ELECTRIFYING MEDICINE

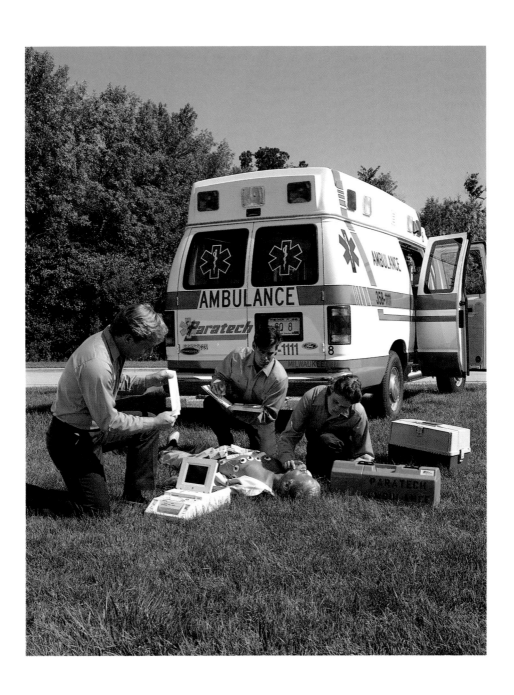

ELECTRIFYING MEDICINE

How Electricity Sparked a Medical Revolution

Brenda L. Himrich
and
Stew Thornley

Lerner Publications Company
Minneapolis

To the Phyllises

The authors would like to extend thanks: to Earl Bakken for generously sharing his time and knowledge; to the employees of Medtronic, Inc., for their assistance; to the staff of The Bakken Library and Museum for their hospitality; to the FES Information Center in Cleveland; and most of all, to our editor, Larry Zwier, for his unwavering encouragement and support.

Library of Congress Cataloging-in-Publication Data

Himrich, Brenda L.
    Electrifying medicine : how electricity sparked a medical
  revolution / by Brenda L. Himrich and Stew Thornley.
      p. cm.
    Includes index.
    ISBN 0-8225-1571-7
    1. Electrotherapeutics—Juvenile literature. I. Thornley, Stew.
  II. Title.
  RM872.H55 1994
  615.8'45—dc20

Manufactured in the United States of America
1 2 3 4 5 6 – I/JR – 00 99 98 97 96 95

CONTENTS

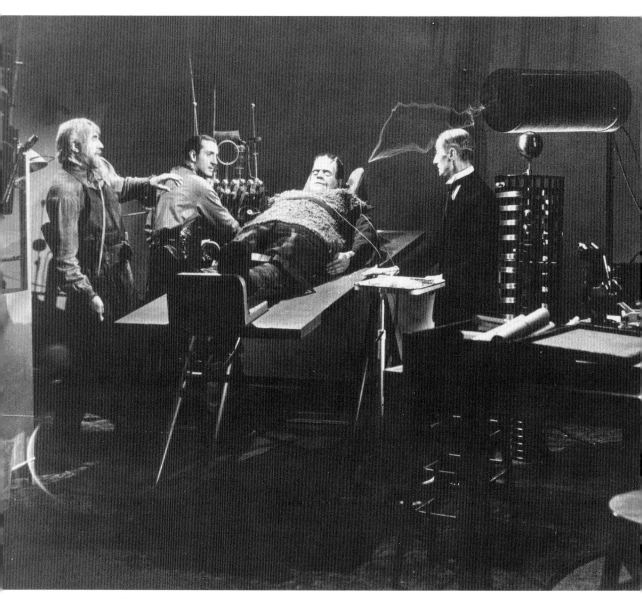

Unleashing electricity into a human body makes one first think of the movie Frankenstein.

INTRODUCTION

A patient lies motionless on a narrow table. A scientist in a white coat approaches, holding a wire in his hand. Touching the wire to the patient's body, he presses a switch to unleash a surge of electricity. The electricity passes into the body of the patient, and the patient slowly begins to be revitalized.

Is this some horror movie? Is the fictional Dr. Frankenstein trying to jolt life into a creature assembled from parts of dead bodies? Hardly. The scientist is a fully qualified doctor in a modern clinic, and the patient is there for a bit of high-tech treatment.

The idea behind Frankenstein's fictional experiment—that electricity could be a ''spark of life'' in the human body—is far from crazy. Even before the early 19th century, when Mary Shelley wrote about Dr. Frankenstein and his experiments, medical scientists knew there was a connection between electricity and life. As more recent medical research has discovered, the human body itself is an electrical system. Chemical reactions taking place constantly throughout the body create electricity that moves from one part of the body to another. And, like any other electrical system, the human body suffers when its currents go awry.

''Life is electricity. Life is defined by electrical movements in the body. When electricity stops moving—that is death.'' Most doctors would agree with this statement by medical-electricity pioneer Earl Bakken. Life and electricity are very closely related. A once-startling medical technique that takes advantage of this connection—sending electricity directly into a patient's body—has become commonplace.

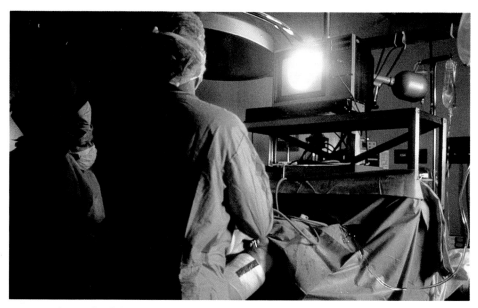

Modern physicians now use a directed flow of electricity as well as electrically powered medical instruments to help heal the body.

Electricity powers countless medical instruments in any modern hospital, clinic, or doctor's office—screens that display a patient's heartbeat, machines that explore the body with X rays, and refrigerators that preserve emergency blood supplies. But electricity also plays a less obvious role in treating illness and saving lives. Electricity can be a kind of medicine itself. Doctors send a flow of electricity directly into a patient's body to stimulate a muscle, to deaden pain, or even to tell a patient's heart how fast to beat. This is what doctors mean by **medical electricity**—electricity used as a treatment for illness or injury.

You are familiar with electricity as some mysterious, powerful force that comes from outlets in the walls of your house and makes machines run. You know that electricity is very dangerous and that you must never touch it. As you have been told ever since you were very young, electricity can kill you. How is it possible for something so dangerous to be produced inside your own body?

Most uses of medical electricity became available only recently. Many others are still experimental and may not be used widely until far into the 21st century—if ever. But simpler medical uses of electricity can be traced back two thousand years, long before anyone understood the electrical nature of the body.

In about A.D. 50, for example, Scribonius Largus, physician to Emperor Claudius of Rome, discovered that the electric torpedo fish—a fish who creates enough electricity inside its body to shock anyone who touches it—could help treat human ailments. Scribonius wrote that ''for any type of gout [an inflammation of the joints], a live black torpedo should, when the pain begins, be placed under the feet. The patient must stand on a moist shore washed by the sea and he should stay like this until his whole foot and leg up to the knee is numb.''

Modern doctors, though they would not ask their patients to stand on sea creatures, would agree that Scribonius had a good idea. Electricity is still used to ease pain, with sophisticated electronic devices doing the fish's job. Electric pain control can even be safer than other treatments. ''Electricity is in many ways better than drugs, since it has a specific location it's going to,'' Earl Bakken has pointed out. ''It doesn't distribute itself throughout the body.'' Electricity can target the pain without causing unwanted side effects, such as sleepiness or an upset stomach.

Pain relief is just one benefit of medical electricity. Low-level electricity from a small machine called a pacemaker can keep a heart beating. Electricity can bring new movement to inactive muscles in a paralyzed arm or leg. Electricity is already helping the deaf hear and the blind see.

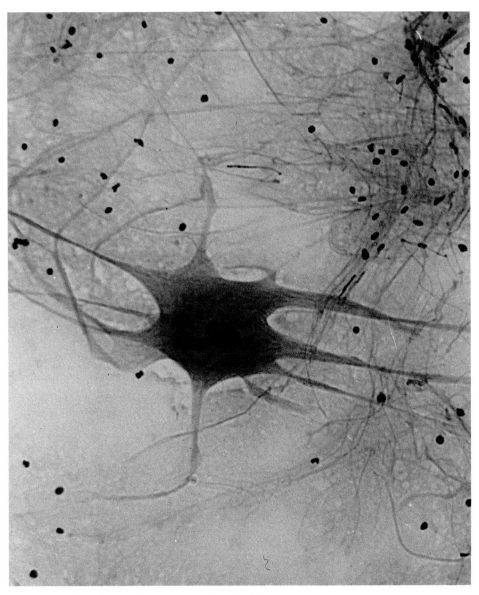

Electricity flows through our bodies from one neuron, or nerve cell, shown here, to another.

CHAPTER
1

THE BODY ELECTRIC

You are surrounded by electricity. The hum of an air conditioner cooling your home is one reminder of electricity at work. Your home may also be heated electrically in the winter. Watching your favorite television show would not be possible without electricity. And think of all the appliances in your kitchen that are powered by electricity. But the most important electrical mechanism in your life is your own body.

It doesn't whir or flash or beep while it's at work, but your body is electrically active every second of your life. A very complex system within your body generates electrical signals, passes them to your muscles, and turns them into actions.

What Is Electricity?

Electricity consists of a flow of tiny particles called electrons. Atoms, which are the building blocks for every substance including air and water, are made up of electrons, protons, and neutrons.

The characteristic that determines how a particle will act when it is near other particles is called charge. The proton has a positive charge, the electron a negative charge, and the neutron a neutral charge—neither positive nor negative. Because the proton and electron have opposite charges, they are attracted to each other. Particles with the same charge move away from one another.

Most atoms have the same number of protons as electrons, so the positive and negative charges in a typical atom balance each other. This balance gives the entire atom a neutral charge. But many atoms can easily gain or lose electrons. If electrons are added to an atom, the atom has a negative charge. If electrons are lost, the atom has a positive charge. These charged atoms, called **ions,** are attracted to other ions that have the opposite charge—positive ions to negative ions and negative ions to positive ions.

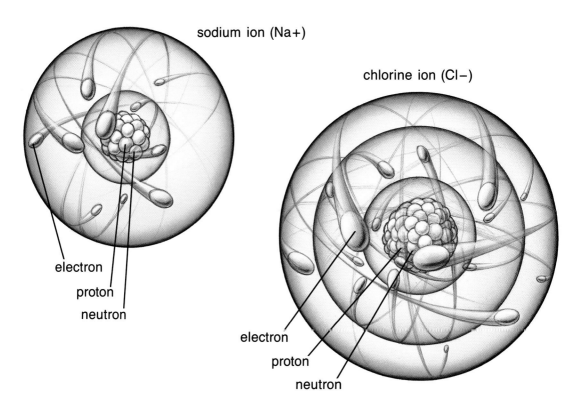

sodium ion (Na+)

chlorine ion (Cl−)

electron

proton

neutron

electron

proton

neutron

Sodium (Na^+) ions, which are missing one electron, and chlorine (Cl^-) ions, which have an extra electron, are found in the fluids in our bodies.

12

When two ions with opposite charges are near one another, each has a chance to become a neutrally charged atom again. The negative ion would become neutral by losing some electrons, and the positive ion would become neutral by gaining some. If enough negative ions together give up electrons that move toward positive ions, a flow of electrons in one direction is created. This flow creates an **electric current**—a flow of charge in a certain direction.

Electricity is what happens when ions come near one another and electrons move from negative ions to positive ions. The ability of electrons to move in a definite direction—to flow in a current—is a basic feature of electricity. Charge and current both help explain how the human body produces electricity and transmits it throughout the body.

Neurons and Electrochemistry

The basic building block in the human electrical system is a spidery cell known as a **neuron.** Neurons make up your brain, your spinal cord, and a network of nerves that carries electrical messages throughout your body. Many of the signals passing from neuron to neuron are directed toward muscles. A set of signals might, for example, be a message from the brain that certain muscles in the arm are supposed to move.

At the center of each neuron is a cell body, where most of the neuron's activity occurs. From there, several extensions called **dendrites** branch out. One longer tubelike structure, called the **axon,** also projects from the cell body. The dendrites can pick up signals from other neurons in the neighborhood. The axon helps carry such signals toward still other neurons or toward muscles and glands. This signal-transmission process is electrochemical—that is, electricity and chemicals both play a role.

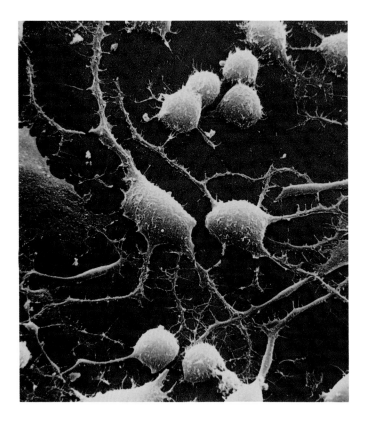

A magnified view of neurons

The attraction between positive and negative ions, as well as the current they can create, is very important in the way neurons work. A neuron that is at rest—not picking up or passing along a message—contains more negative ions than positive. The body fluid surrounding the neuron contains plenty of positive ions of sodium, but these positive ions cannot easily enter the cell. A thin covering of protein called a **membrane** surrounds the neuron and keeps most of the sodium ions out. This creates a big difference in charge between the fluid inside a cell, with its many negative ions, and the fluid outside, dominated by positive ions. If the membrane stopped keeping them outside, the positive ions would be swiftly drawn inside the cell.

When the membrane is stimulated by a message from a nearby neuron, the membrane lets down its guard and allows positive sodium ions to rush into the cell. If enough positive ions enter at enough points, a chain reaction is set in motion. A newly created electrical charge travels quickly through the cell, eventually speeding down the length of the axon.

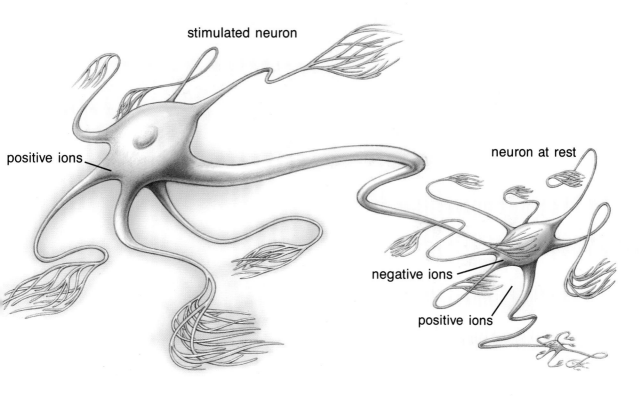

The neuron on the left, having been stimulated, is allowing positive sodium ions to rush into the cell. The neuron on the right is at rest, with negative ions inside and positive ions outside.

15

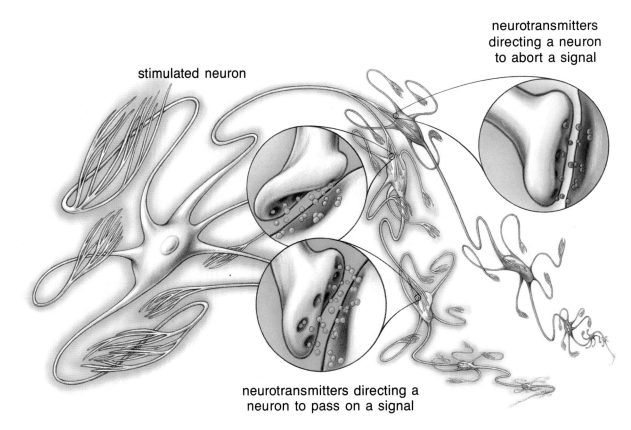

stimulated neuron

neurotransmitters
directing a neuron
to abort a signal

neurotransmitters directing a
neuron to pass on a signal

The neuron on the left directs one neuron, via neurotransmitters, to pick up a signal but tells another neuron to abort the signal.

This charge cannot travel from the axon of one neuron directly to the dendrites of another because a very small gap, called a **synapse,** separates the two neurons. The electrical charge in a human neuron is hardly ever strong enough to jump the synapse. Instead, an impulse that reaches the end of an axon causes the release of chemicals called **neurotransmitters.** These neurotransmitters then spread to the dendrites of other neurons. Some neurotransmitters will cause these neurons to pick up the signal and pass it on. Other neurotransmitters will cause neighboring neurons to abort, or stop, the message. Scientists do not yet know exactly what triggers the release of one type of neurotransmitter instead of another or how a neurotransmitter "knows" which neuron to go to. But the importance of neurotransmitters is clear: They ensure that an impulse travels the proper pathways through the nervous system instead of flashing randomly throughout the body.

Messages from the brain to a muscle will eventually arrive at a group of neurons right next to the target muscle. When the signal gets there, these neurons transmit their messages, not to other neurons, but to the muscle itself. This brings into play another part of the body electric.

Stimulating a Muscle Cell

When most people imagine the body in motion, they think of arms raising, legs stepping, the head nodding, or some other visible movement. But inside the body is another, unseen universe of motion. The heart pumps, lungs inflate, intestines ripple. These countless unseen motions may not be glamorous, but they keep people alive.

Whether a bodily motion is obvious or not, muscles make it possible. Muscles come in three types. Skeletal muscle is connected to bones and makes them move. Smooth muscle makes up such internal organs as the stomach and intestines. Cardiac muscle makes up most of one essential organ, the heart.

A muscle, no matter what type it is, cannot act unless its cells are stimulated. Normally, the stimulation that sets a muscle in motion is a set of electrochemical signals from neurons.

A muscle cell is surrounded by a membrane. Like the membrane surrounding a neuron, this membrane keeps most positive ions out of the cell unless some kind of stimulation—such as a signal from a neuron—causes the membrane to allow positive ions to rush in. The inrush of positive ions gives the inside of the muscle cell a positive charge for a short time. This change in the cell's charge triggers the release, from storage areas inside the cell, of chemicals that make the muscle cell contract. If several muscle cells near one another contract at the same time, the whole muscle contracts and part of the body moves. When the stimulus that led to the contraction is removed, the cell pumps the positive sodium ions out, the cell's chemical balance returns to normal, and the muscle cell relaxes.

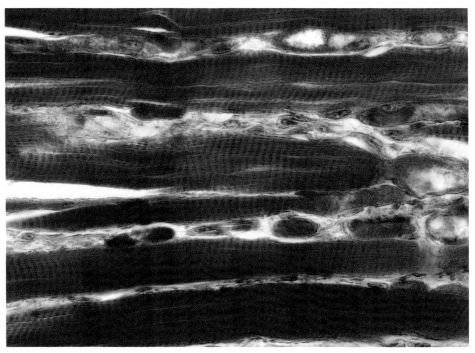

A magnified view of skeletal muscle

Controlling the Signal

One neuron sends signals to another. Neurons communicate with muscles and other bodily tissue. But where do all of these electrical impulses start? And, with so many electrical messages speeding through the body, what directs them all to the right places?

The body's electrochemical messages can be prompted by countless events outside or inside the body. Light might enter the eye and stimulate neurons there. Heat or pressure can stimulate neurons in the skin. Chemicals escaping from an injured internal organ might be sensed by neurons in the area of the injury. One part of the heart—the sinoatrial node—is capable, by itself, of generating electrical signals. So is the brain, in the still-mysterious process known as thought.

No matter how a message gets started, it must be precisely controlled as it moves through the body. The control of these messages is very complex. Although no one can explain exactly how every message is directed along the right path of neurons, the spinal cord and the brain play vital roles in the process.

The **spinal cord** is a cable of neurons that is surrounded and protected by the backbone, or spine. Some of the electrical messages passing among neurons get to their destinations by way of the spinal cord without being routed to the brain. Relatively simple movements—such as the reflexive jerk of a knee tapped by a hammer—usually follow this spinal path. The brain is informed later that the reflex motion has occurred, but the brain is not involved in making it happen.

Other movements of the body result from messages processed in the brain. These messages include many movements that are not consciously thought about. For example, you don't consciously decide to adjust your balance when you stumble. Parts of your brain—having received the message that you are falling—automatically send rapid instructions that set your arms, your legs, and other parts of your body in motion to keep you upright. Other parts of your brain control the movements of your internal organs.

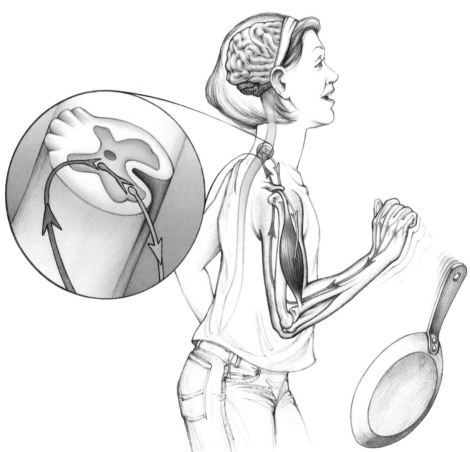

When your hand touches a hot pan, the nerves in your hand send a message to the neurons in your spinal cord. Without going to your brain, a second message speeds back from your spinal cord to the muscles in your hand, and you drop the pan.

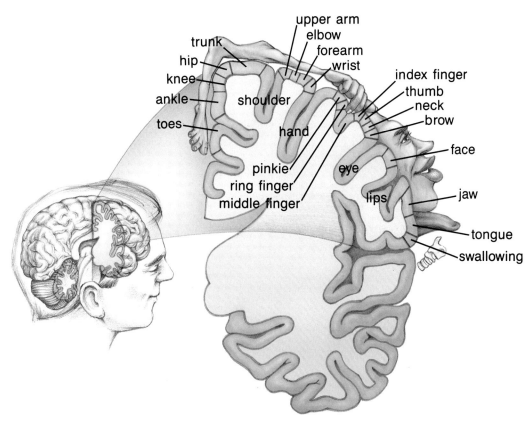

A cross-section of the brain shows the areas of the motor cortex that control different parts of the body.

As it sends out information to control functions throughout the body, the brain acts like an incredibly powerful computer.

In directing many of the body's movements, the brain and the spinal cord work together. A message picked up in some part of the body below the neck is relayed, by way of the spinal cord, to the brain. The brain orders any necessary response and transmits this electrical order through the spinal cord. In this way, the neurons of the spinal cord are like a vital highway leading to and from the brain. If that highway is put out of service, the brain loses its ability to communicate with much of the body.

21

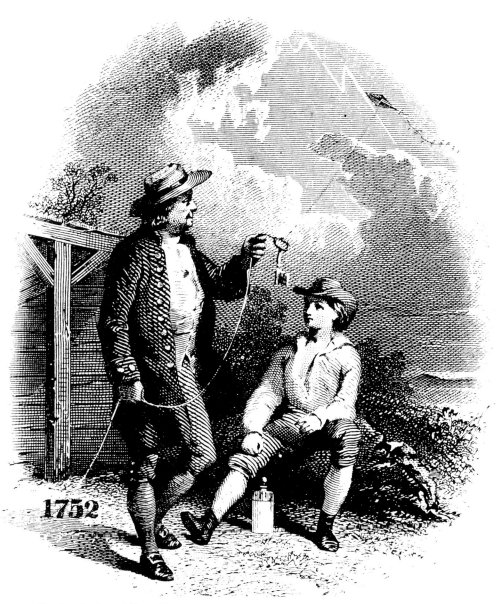

Benjamin Franklin's kite experiment showed that lightning, like other forms of electricity, travels along a conductor toward the ground. Unlike others who tried it, Franklin survived this dangerous experiment.

22

CHAPTER
2

THE CURRENT
OF HISTORY

The doctors of ancient Rome who used electric fish to treat physical ailments knew that their treatment was working, but they didn't know why. At that time, no one knew what electricity was. They could only speculate about what enabled a torpedo fish to relieve pain. One popular guess was that an invisible poison flowed out of the fish and attacked the cause of the pain. Many centuries would pass before scientists could show that an electrical discharge from the fish deserved the credit.

A great awakening to the powers of electricity took place in the 1700s. Generators that produced static electricity—electricity that is not moving in a current—became effective during the 1730s. By 1745 an interesting device called a Leyden jar had been developed. A Leyden jar could store enough static electricity to produce very strong shocks, a feature that medical therapists would learn to use. Still, even though scientists could generate electricity and store it, they knew little about what electricity could do. Then, in the 1750s, an inquisitive colonial American conducted experiments that would greatly advance the study of electricity.

Benjamin Franklin suspected that lightning was electricity. If his idea was correct, lightning, like other forms of electricity, should be able to travel along conductors—objects that can easily carry electricity—toward the ground. His famous kite experiment in 1752, in which he drew a bolt of lightning to a key on a kite string, helped to earn him recognition as one of the world's top authorities on electricity. (Franklin was lucky to survive this dangerous experiment; the next two people who tried it were killed by lightning.) By advancing many helpful ideas about electricity, such as the concept of positive and negative charge, Franklin turned electricity from an almost spiritual mystery into an object of scientific study.

Toys and Frogs

As the secrets of electricity were being discovered, the question became: "What should we do with it?" The earliest answers lay in two fields that seem very different from one another: entertainment and medicine.

During the 18th century, public interest in electricity was soaring, and demonstrations of its use drew large audiences. Electric-powered toys—such as dancing figurines and merry-go-rounds—awed crowds throughout Europe and the Americas. The power of electricity was captivating.

While the crowds applauded and the toys whirled, more serious investigations into electricity's uses were under way. Medical therapy based on electricity seemed like a promising possibility. The effects of electricity on nerves and muscles were demonstrated especially well in separate experiments by two brilliant Italian scientists.

In 1781 Luigi Galvani, a leading medical professor from Bologna, Italy, was studying the relationship between animal tissue and electricity. In one of his experiments, he placed part of a dead frog on a metal hook and hung it from a metal railing. Even though

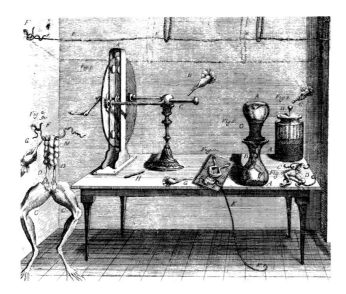

Luigi Galvani's frog experiment convinced him that animal tissue could generate its own electricity.

he did not send any electricity into the dead muscles, they moved. This convinced him that animal tissue could generate its own electricity. A few years later, Galvani's theory of "animal electricity" was disputed by another Italian, Alessandro Volta. Volta argued that the electricity moving the dead frog's muscles resulted from the contact of two pieces of metal—the hook and the railing—not from the animal tissue itself.

The experiments of Galvani, Volta, and others represented the quieter side of 18th-century interest in medical electricity. Less scientific therapists eagerly offered electrical treatment—for a variety of ills and in a variety of doses—to equally eager patients. In one of the milder treatments, an "electric bath," a patient stood or sat on a wooden platform and was connected by a wire or some other conductor to a machine that generated electricity. As patients bathed in the "electric fluid"—actually a low charge of electricity that traveled throughout the body—they felt drowsy, calm,

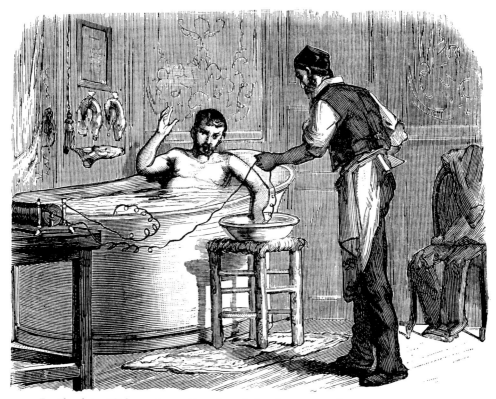

In the late 19th century, the electric bath was used to treat severe headaches and muscle pains.

and pain-free. These baths were used well into the 20th century to treat severe headaches, muscle pains, and other ailments. Did electric baths really improve anyone's health? It's hard to say, because they were not used or tested very scientifically. In any case, they probably didn't hurt anyone, because the electricity they used was very weak.

In mild doses like those of an electric bath, electricity seemed like a quick, clean, and relatively painless treatment. It was obviously better than much of the crude, painful surgery practiced

26

in the 18th and 19th centuries. In some cases, it was even better than chemical medicine. A physician named T. Gale, in his 1802 book *Electricity or Ethereal Fire,* claimed that electric shocks had restored his own health. He also complained that doctors prescribed artificial drugs to treat many ailments instead of using a natural treatment—electricity. Its gentle reputation in these early days gave electrical medicine some influential supporters, including the religious leader John Wesley, the founder of the Methodist Church.

Doctors in the 18th and 19th centuries also had some generally harmless (and sometimes effective) ways of using electricity to treat muscles. Because electrical shocks can make muscles twitch—even muscles that cannot be moved voluntarily—low doses of electricity were used as early as 1747 to exercise weak or paralyzed muscles. Electrical current was also used to reduce muscle spasms—unwanted and uncontrollable movements of a muscle.

Electroquackery

Not all electrical discoveries were valid, and many medical treatments were pure nonsense. There was no shortage of people trying to make a little money from the public's fascination with electricity. Disreputable fakers known as quacks offered electrical therapy that looked impressive but really had no helpful medical effect.

One slightly strange device was the electric belt, which was prescribed for all types of diseases. The first electric belt, invented in 1801, was made up of small square plates of zinc connected by links of copper. The inventor recommended this current-emitting belt for relief of "a constant pain in the small of the back and loins." A later version of the belt, produced by the Pulvermacher Galvanic Company, consisted of several wooden cylinders

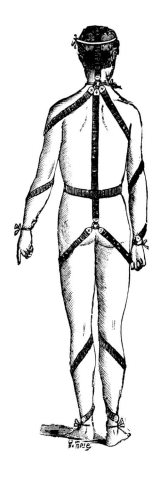

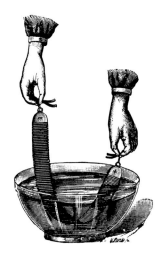

This advertisement shows how a patient would use an electric belt to relieve pain.

filled with zinc and copper wires and joined in a series on a flexible belt. Before putting on this belt, the wearer had to soak it in vinegar, to increase its ability to carry electricity. The belt's manufacturers claimed that it would cure "all nervous, chronic, and functional diseases." Other wearable electrical devices—corsets, rings, shoe inserts—were also for sale.

These outlandish gadgets, however, were not nearly as flaky as a device, called the I-ON-A-CO, invented in 1926 by a Californian named Gaylord Wilshire. A clever businessperson with no known medical background, Wilshire claimed to have discovered a way of using electricity "for the cure of human ailments." The I-ON-A-CO was a coil 18 inches in diameter, which was worn around the body. It was made of insulated wire and had a plug that could be inserted into any household electric socket.

Wilshire used full-page newspaper advertisements to proclaim how wondrous his invention was. The I-ON-A-CO, he claimed, would not only cure diseases but also make the user beautiful "quickly, neatly, and without pain." The American Medical Association (AMA) compared the I-ON-A-CO's therapeutic value to that of the "left hind foot of a rabbit caught in a churchyard in the dark of the moon." Because of investigations by the AMA, Wilshire's I-ON-A-CO was quickly discredited—but not before its inventor had made a lot of money by selling it.

Swings in Popularity

Since the 18th century, the popularity of electrical medicine has had many ups and downs. A pattern seemed to develop: great interest in medical electricity late in one century, then a steep decline early in the next. Interest in electrotherapy was strong in the final years of the 1700s, but it decreased near the beginning of the 19th century. Most likely, all the quacks doing business at that time had given medical electricity a bad reputation. But electrical therapy eventually made a comeback, rising to great popularity late in the 19th century.

By the early 20th century, large amounts of electricity were being generated to light streets, to power industrial machinery, and even to be sent directly into private homes. Most people learned that electricity could kill, so a fear of electrical treatments developed. After the middle of the 20th century, however, this fear of electricity faded. The effects of electricity on the body once again became the subject of great interest and research. In the closing years of the 20th century, electricity has finally found a permanent place in the treatment of human ailments.

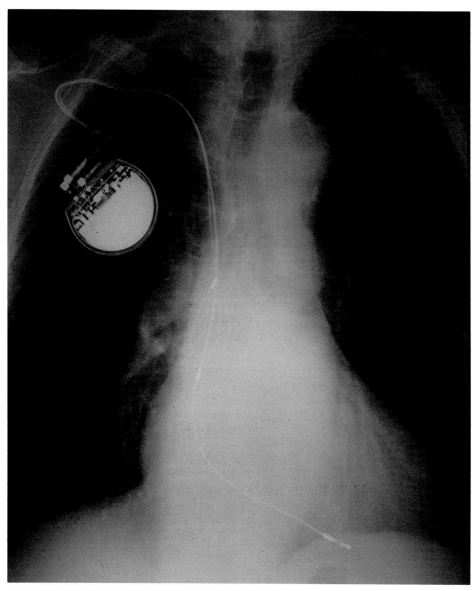

When people's hearts don't beat regularly, pacemakers are implanted in their chests. This X ray shows the pacemaker.

CHAPTER
3

A CHARGE
TO THE HEART

Inside your body is a pump. It is barely larger than a baseball and weighs only about 10 ounces. Yet this tiny pump is strong enough to move blood throughout your body every minute of your life. It operates in your chest at the center of a complicated network of blood-carrying tubes. This hardworking organ is your heart.

To understand some of what your heart goes through, place a tennis ball in your hand, squeeze it, and then relax your grip. Squeeze and relax again. Then do it faster, until you go through a squeeze-and-relax cycle once per second. This is essentially what your heart does, but even a little bit faster. On an average of 72 times a minute, it contracts and then relaxes.

How long could you keep squeezing that tennis ball before tiring? Within a few minutes, you'd probably be ready to put the ball down. Your heart, however, keeps on going—without rest—throughout your lifetime. If it didn't, your blood would stop moving. Without the important nutrients and oxygen that blood carries, your other organs could not function. You would die. What keeps the heart going? And, just as importantly, what regulates the rhythm of its beat? Electricity is the answer.

The heart is made up almost entirely of muscle cells, which can stretch and contract just like other muscle cells. The heart's contractions—heartbeats—propel blood through the body, and electrical impulses are responsible for making sure that the heart beats with the proper rhythm. These impulses are generated in the heart itself by a group of heart cells called the **sinoatrial (SA) node.**

To cause a full heartbeat, a message from the SA node has to be conducted throughout the heart. Since there are no nerves in the heart, the heart muscle itself and certain specialized fibers carry this impulse. First the message tells muscle cells in the **atriums**—two of the heart's four chambers—to contract. Then the impulse travels through the heart muscle to a message center called the **atrioventricular (AV) node,** located between the right atrium and the heart's other two chambers, the **ventricles.** After pausing briefly in the AV node, the impulse moves through conducting fibers and directs the ventricles to contract.

The timing of the electrical impulse is critical. If the timing is off, the atriums and ventricles will not contract in the proper sequence. Someone whose heartbeat is not properly timed might feel weak, confused, or even dizzy enough to faint. The heart needs not only a dose of electricity, but a finely timed one.

The normal pace of the heartbeat varies a little from person to person. Also, each person's heart beats more rapidly at some times than at others. Exercising, for example, will cause your heart to contract and relax more rapidly than when you are at rest. For most people, whether they are resting or working up a sweat, the SA node sets an appropriate pace. But, like any other electrical system, the heart's rhythmic system does not always function properly. Some people have heart-rhythm problems from the time of birth. The pace of the heart can be thrown off by damage from a heart attack or by repairs made during heart surgery. Even the normal aging process can take its toll on the heart.

Electricity has been extremely valuable in treating two very different irregularities in the heart's rhythm. In one, the heart must have outside electrical help to maintain any beat at all. In the other, electrical current is used to keep the heart from beating out of control.

Artificial Pacing

When someone's heart has trouble keeping a beat, he or she may be given a **pacemaker,** a tiny electrical device inserted in the body to artificially regulate the beat of the heart. In effect, a pacemaker takes over for a malfunctioning SA or AV node. Pacemakers have become so common that, in 1993, about 1.5 million Americans had artificial pacemakers. Pacemaker wearers have ranged in age from less than one day old to 115 years old. Because tiny modern pacemakers operate unseen within the user's body—and because people who have them can lead very active lives—it's not often easy to tell someone who has one from someone who doesn't.

A crude device often regarded as the first pacemaker was used in the 1930s by a doctor named Albert S. Hyman. In 1952, Dr. Paul M. Zoll introduced an improved pacemaker that made artificial pacing more practical. Early pacemakers, however, were bulky units that had to remain outside the body. Not only that, but users of the early pacemaker experienced a painful stinging where the pacemaker's electrodes (the parts that come into contact with the body and deliver the current) touched their skin. The development of pacemakers took a major step forward in 1957—thanks to a group of babies at the University of Minnesota Hospital in Minneapolis.

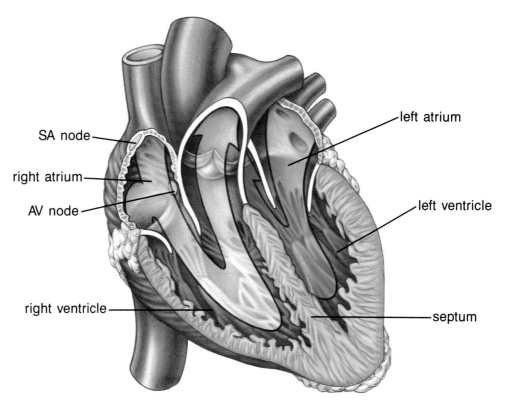

The heart's SA and AV nodes time the heartbeat, which regulates the flow of oxygenated blood from the lungs to the rest of the body and the flow of oxygen-poor blood to the lungs.

Blue Babies

It is not highly unusual for babies to be born with an opening in the septum, a wall of muscle that separates the right and left ventricles of the heart. Normally, the hole will gradually close on its own. In the hearts of some babies, however, the opening remains. As a result, oxygen-poor blood, which is bluish in color, comes from the right side of the heart and mixes with the red oxygen-rich blood in the left part. As this mixture of blood flows through the body, it leaves the babies' skin with a bluish tint. For this reason, the infants are known as "blue babies."

Dr. C. Walton Lillehei, a heart surgeon at the University of Minnesota, specialized in treating blue babies. He was able to close the hole in the septum by sewing a patch over it. This solved the problem of the unwanted mixing of blood, but it created a new difficulty for some of the babies. In about 20 percent of the babies, the sutures, or stitches, that held the patch in place interfered with the electrical conduction in the heart. Artificial pacemakers were needed to control the heartbeats of these babies.

With the help of other doctors at the hospital, Lillehei developed

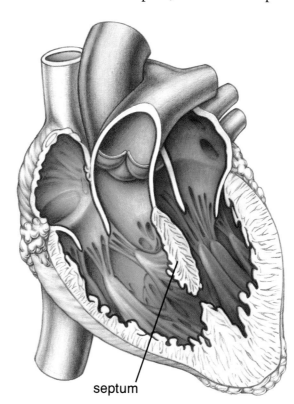

An opening in the heart's septum allows blue oxygen-poor blood to mix with red oxygen-rich blood.

septum

a pacemaker especially for the babies, one that sent a mild electrical current through wires attached directly to the babies' hearts. But these pacemakers, like earlier versions, needed an external power source. They had to be plugged into electrical outlets at the hospital.

In the summer of 1957, a violent thunderstorm left the hospital without electricity for several hours. Emergency generators were

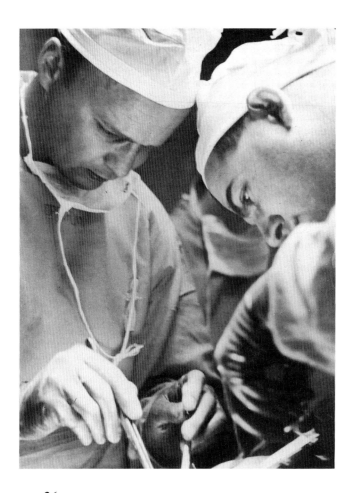

Dr. C. Walton Lillehei, right, performs surgery.

36

turned on to supply power to equipment in the operating rooms. But the rooms for patients who had already come out of surgery—including the blue babies—had no backup supply. Without artificial heart pacing, one of the blue babies died.

Dr. Lillehei was disturbed by this death. He knew that the tragedy could have been avoided if the pacemakers had been battery-powered, independent of the usual power supply. At that time, an electronics technician named Earl Bakken was selling equipment to the university hospital. Lillehei asked Bakken if an internally powered pacemaker were possible.

Bakken knew that a pacemaker required very little power—so little that a small battery could supply it. The challenge was to produce a rhythmic pulse of power that could be timed just right. Paging through an electronics magazine, Bakken discovered a design for an electronic system that produced a steady but adjustable pulse. Within a few weeks, Bakken had adapted this design to power a pacemaker.

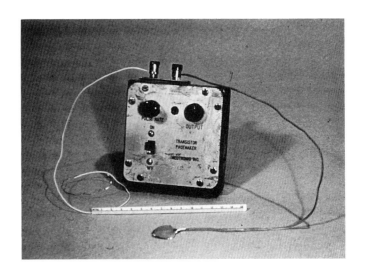

Bakken's first pacemaker. The entire design fits inside a small plastic box.

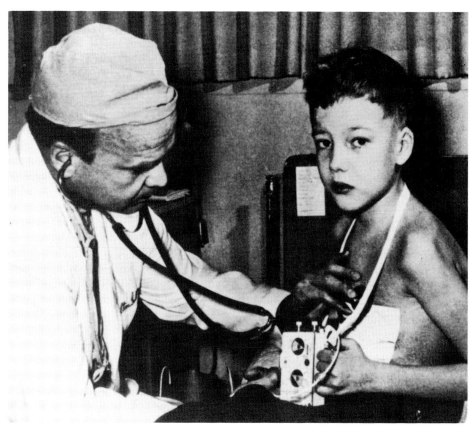

Dr. C. Walton Lillehei, left, examines David Williams, a young cardiac patient wearing an external pacemaker of the type invented by Earl Bakken.

Bakken's invention was just what Dr. Lillehei wanted—a self-powered pacemaker. After the University of Minnesota had successfully tested the new pacemaker on laboratory animals, Lillehei began using the units on the babies under his care. He strapped the devices to their chests and connected the electrodes to their hearts. The pacemakers worked.

The 1957 pacemaker was not perfect. The unit was smaller than in earlier models, but it was still large. And it was outside the patient's body. A pacemaker user had to carry a little box along wherever he or she went. Within a few years, however, another milestone was reached.

In upstate New York, a surgeon named William Chardack and an electrical engineer named Wilson Greatbatch worked together to develop a battery-operated pacemaker small enough to fit inside the body. In 1960 Dr. Chardack successfully implanted a pacemaker in a human body. The user finally enjoyed the freedom of a heart that depended on nothing outside his or her own chest. Later that year, Chardack and Greatbatch signed a contract with a Minneapolis company to produce their implantable pulse generator. The company, called Medtronic, had been founded by Earl Bakken, the technician who had helped Dr. Lillehei and the blue babies.

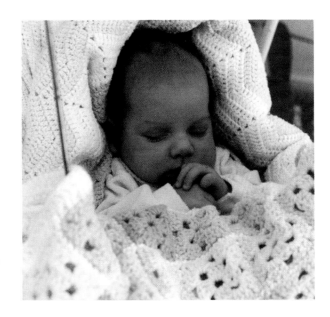

Surgeons will close the hole in this blue baby's septum and implant a pacemaker to regulate his heartbeat.

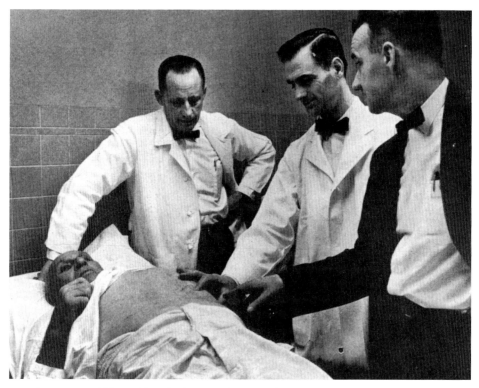

Doctors William Chardack, standing at left, and Andrew Gage, center, implanted the first self-contained, self-powered pacemaker for Frank Henefelt, 77, on April 18, 1960. William Greatbatch, right, designed and built the unit.

Changing the Beat

Improvements in size and power supply continued, but other major developments also helped make pacemakers more practical. The first pacemakers caused the heart to beat at a continuous, fixed rate. Pacing of this type is called **asynchronous pacing.** Asynchronous pacemakers worked, but unlike the heart's natural system, they did not allow the heartbeat to adjust to the body's activity level by quickening or slowing down. Also, they pulsed away all the time, whether the heart needed their signals or not.

Later, a new type of pacemaker was developed. It still maintained a continuous minimum heart rate, but it clicked into action only when needed—if the heart either stopped beating or beat slower than the pacemaker's fixed rate. At other times, the pacemaker stayed quietly ready, conserving its power. Because this type of pacemaker can sense when it is needed, the system is called **demand pacing.**

The latest generation of pacemakers can vary the heart rate in response to bodily needs. For example, these pacemakers increase the heart rate during physical activity and reduce it when the body is at rest. This ability to vary the heart rate imitates the normal operation of a healthy heart. These **rate-responsive pacemakers** can tell—by sensing such bodily conditions as increased muscle activity, faster breathing, or changes in body temperature—that a change in the heart rate is needed. The pacemaker then adjusts the timing of the electrical pulses it emits.

Pacemaker Design

All pacemakers have three basic parts: a pulse generator, a pacing lead, and an electrode. The pulse generator produces an electric signal; the lead carries this signal to the heart; the electrode provides the electrical connection to the heart.

The pulse generator consists of a tiny battery and some miniature electronic circuitry inside a small metal container. The pacemaker's battery, like any ordinary battery, supplies energy. But unlike the batteries in a flashlight or a watch, a pacemaker's battery, planted inside the user's body, cannot easily be changed. For that reason, pacemaker batteries are specially designed to last for a long time—10 years is not unusual—and are permanently sealed inside the pulse generator. If the battery gets weak (at which time the user's heart-beat might become slightly irregular) the user goes into surgery to have the whole pulse generator, not just the battery, replaced.

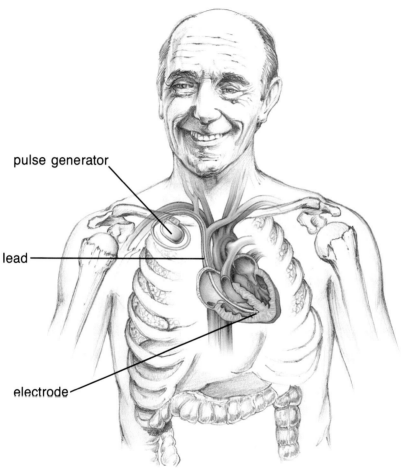

pulse generator

lead

electrode

A pacemaker, implanted in a person's body, has three parts: a pulse generator to produce the electrical signal, a pacing lead to carry the signal to the heart, and an electrode to make the electrical connection to the heart.

The lead is an insulated wire that goes from the pulse generator to the heart. Sometimes, the pulse generator is implanted quite far from the heart—just above the waist at one side of the body, for example—so the lead has to be not only long but also flexible enough to withstand the body's twisting and bending. At the tip of the lead is a metal piece that can be planted in or on the heart. This is the electrode, which delivers the electrical energy to the heart. Electric pulses come through this electrode to stimulate the surrounding heart tissue and cause the heart to beat. In demand-

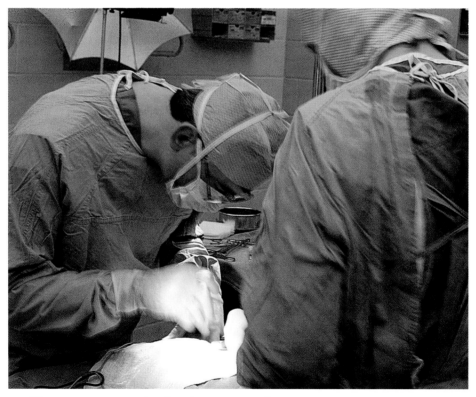

These surgeons are implanting a pacemaker.

pacing systems, the electrode senses the heart's natural activity and transmits this information back to the pulse generator.

Pacemakers can be inserted into the body in two different ways. Usually, a lead is slipped into a vein in the upper chest and is then threaded through the vein to the right side of the heart. The electrode from the lead will then rest directly against the inner wall of the heart. This type of insertion is called a transvenous implant. The other type of implant is called an epicardial—"on the heart"—implant. The chest is opened in surgery, and the electrode is attached directly to the heart muscle. In both types of implant, the pulse generator is placed under the skin in either the upper chest or the lower abdomen—wherever it will be most comfortable for the patient and best protected from damage. Implanting a pacemaker used to require a long and involved operation, but now the necessary surgery usually takes less than an hour.

Different types of pacemakers treat different types of problems. Patients with damage to the SA node need stimulation in only one chamber of the heart. These patients will probably use a single-chamber pacemaker, which has a single lead wire going to one chamber of the heart, usually a ventricle. A patient who has a healthy SA node but has serious problems at the AV node will probably need a dual-chamber pacemaker. This type of pacemaker has two leads, one going to the right atrium and the other to a ventricle. The pacemaker will ensure that the atrium contracts first and, after a short pause, the ventricle contracts.

Pacemakers have greatly increased the life expectancy of people with heart-rhythm problems. Lightweight metals and advanced electronic circuitry have made pacemakers smaller, lighter, and more streamlined. The more than 2.5 million people who have had pacemaker implants have led fuller, more active lives despite their heart problems.

Defibrillation

Another disorder of the heart's rhythm, one too severe for a pacemaker to remedy, is **ventricular fibrillation.** In fibrillation, a person's heart suddenly races out of control, quivering rather than pumping. The left ventricle, which is the heart's main pumping chamber, suddenly stops beating regularly and goes into a state of uncontrolled fluttering.

When this happens, the victim must receive a powerful electric shock to the chest to jolt the fibrillating heart back to normal. Unless this shock comes within eight minutes of the onset of fibrillation, the victim will probably die.

You may have seen television dramas in which emergency-room doctors give a patient enough electricity to make his or her unconscious body jump suddenly. Scenes like this depict doctors trying to defibrillate a patient's heart by applying a huge surge of electric power. The electric jolt is enormous. It can range from 3,000 to 5,000 volts, vastly stronger than a pacemaker's mild 5-volt shock. A **defibrillator** is the machine that produces this lifesaving shock. It contains a pair of paddles that are placed on the victim's chest to deliver the shock to the heart.

Defibrillators are expensive and dangerous to use. Only trained medical personnel, who usually are not on the scene when an attack of fibrillation occurs, are likely to have a defibrillator. Their speed in arriving with one of these devices can mean the difference between life and death. Too often, they cannot arrive fast enough. Hundreds of thousands of people die each year from ventricular fibrillation because help doesn't arrive in time. To solve this problem, efforts are underway to make defibrillators available for home and office use by people who are not medical professionals.

Computers automate these new types of defibrillators so that a nonprofessional operator does not have to make risky decisions.

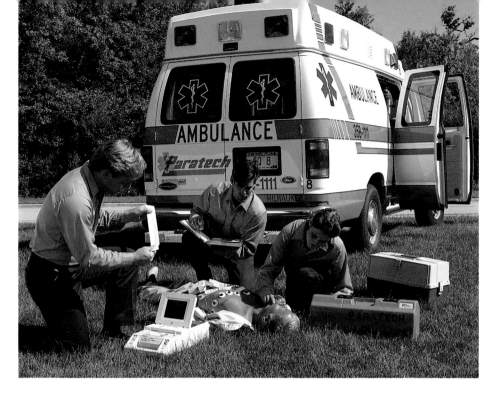

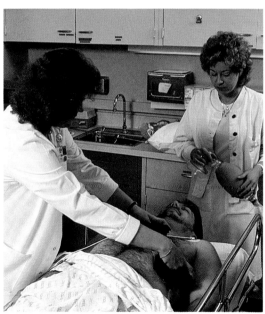

Paramedics, above, and
medical personnel in
emergency rooms, left, are
trained to use defibrillators.
They save many lives, but
computerized defibrillators
used by nonprofessionals
could save many more
people whose hearts
suddenly race out
of control.

The operator can place a pair of electrodes on the victim's chest and allow the defibrillator to analyze the heartbeat. An electric jolt is automatically delivered if it is needed. As the device continues to reassess the heart's condition, it delivers more shocks if they are necessary. It also displays messages that tell the operator what steps to take next. Such machines have been built, but they have to be tested further before they can be made available to the public.

But a different kind of new technology—implantable defibrillators—already makes defibrillation quickly available. People who have a high risk of rhythm disorders—for example, people who have suffered heart attacks or have had episodes of fibrillation in the past—can benefit greatly from such devices. With an implant, they no longer have to worry about fibrillation attacks when no one is around to help them. An implanted defibrillator is always available and ready to go to work immediately. Like a pacemaker, an implanted defibrillator is battery-powered and monitors the heart's electrical discharges. If it senses the beginning of fibrillation, it sends the heart a shock, or several shocks, until the rhythm disturbances stop.

Defibrillators, like pacemakers, have helped people with heart-rhythm problems live longer and enjoy life more. As medical technology develops, making such devices more readily available, defibrillators will play an even greater role in the ability of medical electricity to extend life.

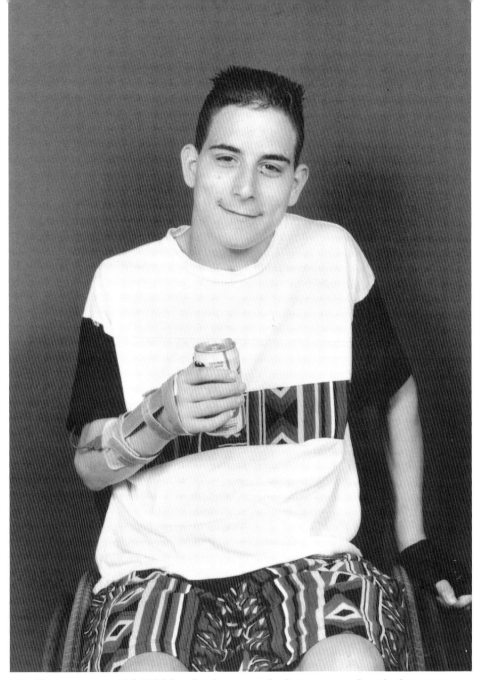

Fourteen-year-old Micki, who has paraplegia, uses an electrical system that stimulates his muscles to move so he can drink from a soda can.

CHAPTER
4

MUSCLE POWER

You are thirsty, so you stand up, walk into the kitchen, and pull open the refrigerator door. You bend over and reach for a can of soda pop on the bottom shelf. You pick up the can, then you stand up straight again, close the door, and use your index finger to flip open the can's pop-top. Bending your arm, you lift the can and tilt it so the cool drink flows into your open mouth.

In trying to quench your thirst, you performed many complex movements—involving your arms, legs, fingers, knees, knuckles, back, neck, and mouth—without even being aware of them. Each of these movements, even a twitch of your mouth or a blink of your eye, was possible because your muscles did what your brain ordered them to do. You might not have been conscious of each move you made, but your brain was busy all the time sending messages to your muscles.

How could the muscles in your hands, arms, and legs get messages from your brain? Your body's electrical system made it possible. Because your nerves were properly conducting electrical signals to your muscles, you were able to leave your chair in the living room and pour a cool drink down your throat. Electricity even allowed you to taste the drink, to know that it was cold, and to enjoy the feel of the bubbles as you swallowed.

Disrupted Pathways

All this happens when the nervous system operates normally. An injury or serious disease, however, might disrupt the communication between brain and muscle. A damaged nervous system will not transmit messages properly, so the body cannot respond to commands from the brain.

In some cases, brain-muscle communication is interrupted because of an injury to the brain—damage that can come from many causes. Someone might suffer a severe blow to the head. A stroke might result in a massive die-off of cells because blood has stopped flowing to a certain area of the brain. A virus might cause encephalitis (a severe swelling of the brain) that could damage brain cells. But brain damage does not underlie every failure of communication between brain and muscle. The root of the problem might be some injury or disease that has damaged the spinal cord.

The human spinal cord, a complex bundle of nerve cells, is the superhighway of nerve paths. Extending from the base of the brain to just below the middle of the back, the spinal cord carries all of the electrical signals that control the muscles from neck to toe. The delicate spinal cord is protected by the backbone, or spine—a column of sturdy, tubular bones called vertebrae. Still, the spine can provide only so much protection. A severe blow or shock to the backbone, perhaps from an automobile accident or a head-first dive into shallow water, can be enough to damage the spinal cord. A severe injury to the spinal cord can cause irreversible damage that may result in paralysis, an inability to move certain muscles.

Injuries to the spinal cord occur approximately 8,000 times a year in the United States. Perhaps as many as 500,000 Americans have suffered a spinal-cord injury that has left them with some

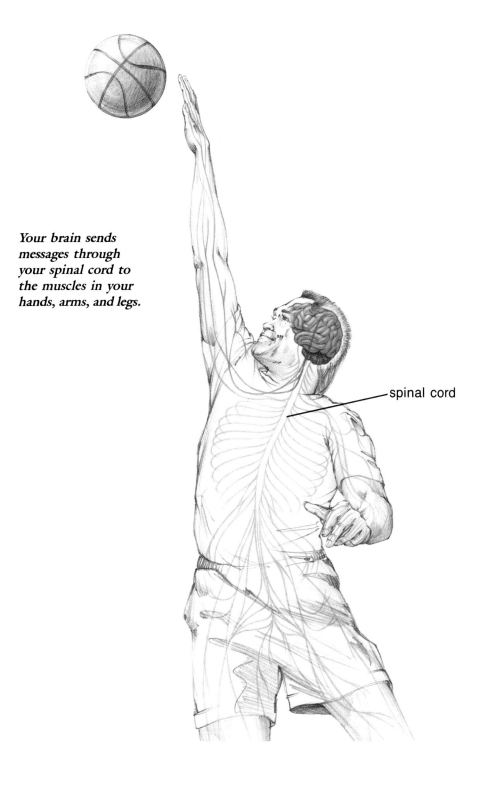

*Your brain sends
messages through
your spinal cord to
the muscles in your
hands, arms, and legs.*

spinal cord

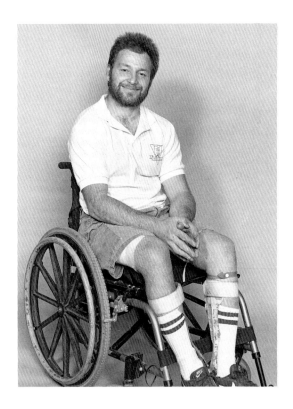

People with severe injuries to their spinal cord can become paralyzed.

form of paralysis. Other spinal-cord injuries stop short of causing paralysis, merely weakening the muscles.

The closer a spinal-cord injury is to a patient's head, the more muscles are likely to be paralyzed. If an injury occurs near the 7 highest vertebrae—the cervical vertebrae—the entire body from the neck down, including the arms, may be paralyzed. This paralysis is known as quadriplegia. Damage to the cord in the area of the next 12 vertebrae—the thoracic vertebrae—can result in paraplegia, paralysis of the legs and lower body. Besides making movements in parts of the body impossible, spinal injuries cut off all feeling in the immobile part of the body.

Until the end of World War I, serious spinal-cord injury did not normally paralyze people. It usually killed them. Since then, advances in medicine and treatment have given those who have suffered such injuries a much greater chance of survival. Many of these survivors, however, remain paralyzed—some very severely—for the rest of their lives. To victims of spinal-cord injury, many of whom were young and healthy before the injury, the prospect of spending the rest of their lives unable to walk or even move their hands can be devastating.

For some people with paralysis, however, electric current offers a glimmer of hope that they might regain limited use of some muscles. The treatments are new, the gains are small, and researchers stress that electricity cannot cure paralysis. Still, even small gains in motor function—the ability to move parts of one's body—can make a big difference to a person with a spinal-cord injury or disease. Since the 1960s, the use of electricity in treating paralysis has been an important focus of research.

Restoring Movement

One of the early breakthroughs took place in 1960 when a researcher named Adrian Kantrowitz attached electrodes to the skin of a patient with paraplegia. When the current was turned on, electricity stimulated certain nerves in the patient's buttocks, thereby causing some muscles to contract. When enough of the right muscles had been stimulated, the patient was eventually able to straighten his knees and even stand up.

Other research groups, building on Kantrowitz's early success, have developed more sophisticated electrical treatments for paralyzed muscles. Some of these treatments are dependable and already in use. Others are still experimental and are being used only in laboratories. Some treatments are relatively simple, using

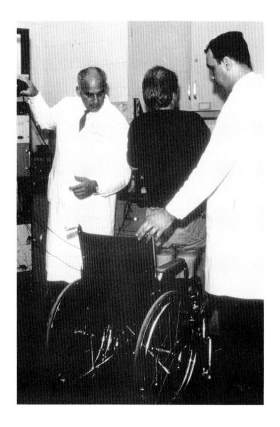

Adrian Kantrowitz, left, *experiments with ways to control the limb movements of a patient with paraplegia.*

electrodes that can be easily attached to a patient's skin. Others require complicated surgery to implant electrodes within the body. None of these treatments can cure spinal injuries. Instead, they offer a way for the patient to bypass the damaged spine while sending electrical signals to muscles.

To use any electrical muscle-stimulation system, the user makes a small movement with an active muscle—perhaps the shrug of a shoulder or a slight hand motion—to turn an electric signal on or off. Different sequences of signals indicate which part of the body a user wants to move. A computer worn on the user's belt then interprets these messages and sends electrical impulses to electrodes planted on or near the muscles that need to be moved. Current from the electrodes stimulates the muscles, causing them to contract. After all these electrical signals have completed their journeys, a person with quadriplegia may be able to grasp and lift a cup, or a person with paraplegia may be able to control enough of the lower body to stand or even walk a little.

An electric current that helps a body part do its job, or function, is called **functional electrical stimulation.** Not all electrical therapy helps body parts function. Electrical current that relieves pain, for example, is a form of ''nonfunctional'' stimulation.

A functional current that helps skeletal muscles move is **functional neuromuscular stimulation (FNS).** FNS works by stimulating neurons, not by directly stimulating muscle cells. The

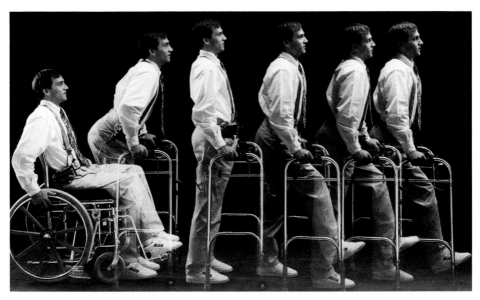

An FNS system helps a patient with paraplegia to stand and walk.

current from outside the body stimulates neurons, which then activate the muscle cells. Even though a current of electricity applied directly to muscles can cause them to contract, muscles stimulated in this way tire quickly. Sending the current through nerves to muscles is the only practical way to help patients move.

Because it needs to work through healthy nerves, FNS can only help patients with upper motor neuron damage. In these cases, the muscles and the neurons that connect directly to them are healthy, but they are not receiving signals from the brain because neurons farther up in the spinal cord have been damaged. FNS is able to bypass these damaged spinal neurons and send electricity through other healthy neurons to muscles.

Unfortunately, FNS cannot help a patient with lower motor neuron damage—that is, with damage to the neurons connected directly to the muscles. When these neurons die, electrical current loses its route into the muscle cells. The muscle cells that the neurons once served, now deprived of stimulation, get smaller. Some even die and disappear.

Successes and Limits

Electrical stimulation has helped some paralyzed patients to both stand and walk. In the mid-1980s, a team led by Dr. E. Byron Marsolais helped two patients with paraplegia at the Cleveland Veterans Administration Medical Center to walk more than 400 feet while using a rolling walker for support and balance. Since then, one of the patients has walked more than 700 feet and has been able to walk up and down stairs while using hand railings.

Other systems are helping people with quadriplegia to move some parts of their upper bodies and arms. Using stimulation, the patients can feed themselves, comb their own hair, and perform other basic daily tasks for themselves. Other accomplishments

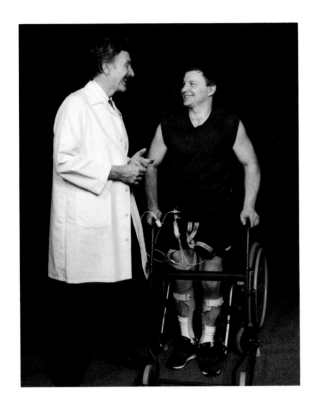

Dr. E. Byron Marsolais jokes with a patient.

such as writing a letter, turning a doorknob, or pushing a remote-control button to change a channel are also possible for people with quadriplegia. FNS systems have also helped people with paralysis to do needlepoint, hold a cue stick, and play slot machines.

James Jatich has benefited from such a system. At the age of 28, Jatich was injured in a diving accident. Besides being completely paralyzed below the waist, he had only very limited use of his arms and hands. Then an electrical-stimulation system enabled Jatich to do some simple things that he had assumed he would never do again. The system used by Jatich is a prototype—the first usable model of a system that might be produced in greater numbers later. It has a pair of microprocessors (parts of a computer that sort information). The first one activates when Jatich sends it a signal by shrugging his shoulder. The second one relays the signal to a radio transmitter. This sends an electric pulse through wires to electrodes implanted in his hand muscles, which then contract. By allowing him to grasp things, the system has enabled Jatich to write letters and feed himself.

Despite a few successes, medical electricity has not yet moved many skeletal muscles in useful ways. Since electricity did so much so quickly for heart patients, high hopes were pinned on FNS. The desire for a quick electrical miracle in stimulating muscles other

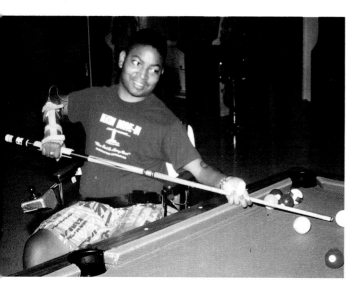

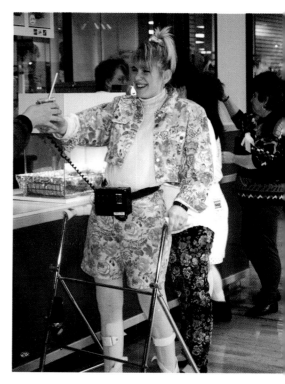

Rico, left, *can play pool with an FNS system. He grips the cue by shrugging his opposite shoulder. Karen,* right, *uses an FNS system to walk around the mall. She controls her stepping with a switch slipped around her finger.*

than the heart is understandable but unrealistic. A leg movement or a handshake involves far more movement than a heartbeat does. A single electrical pulse can cause the heart to beat, but a bewildering network of coordinated signals lies behind every drink from a can of soda pop. Even the best computer programs for sending messages to muscles do not come close to copying the body's natural flow of information.

Another problem for FNS users is the difficulty of knowing when their movements have gone far enough. A healthy nervous system allows a person to react instantly to his or her surroundings. If you take a step, you know that your step is complete when you feel your foot touch the floor. If you reach for a cup, you know you have reached far enough when you feel the cup with your fingers. In other words, you get feedback that tells you how successful your movements have been. But how can someone who relies on FNS feel that her foot is on the ground, or know when his grasp is tight enough to pick up an object? This is not easy. The same injury that interfered with messages from the brain to the muscle will prevent touch-related messages from being relayed back to the brain. Without this feedback, patients cannot efficiently control the movement that FNS makes possible. So far, research has not produced many implantable touch simulators, sensors that could provide this important feedback. Efforts to develop better touch sensors are an important part of muscle-stimulation research.

Overall, electrical stimulation of paralyzed muscles is still an infant science. So far, the idea of independent movement, with FNS totally replacing an attendant or a wheelchair, is still just a dream. But FNS has already meant greater independence for some people. To someone who thought she would never again pour herself a cold drink, even this little taste of freedom can be exhilarating.

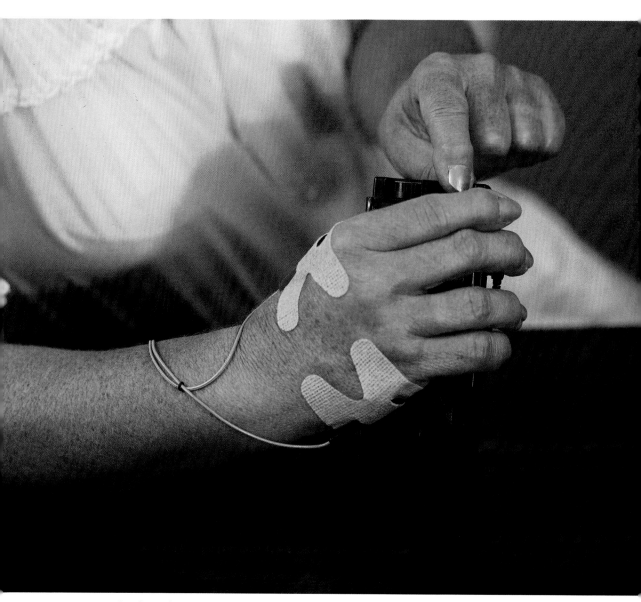

Surface electrodes on the skin deliver electricity to a part of the body suffering from chronic pain.

60

CHAPTER
5

ELECTRICITY AND PAIN MANAGEMENT

Picture yourself in a doctor's office for a routine checkup. The doctor tells you that you need a flu vaccination to keep from getting sick. You're trying to stay calm, but you get a little nervous when you see the needle. The doctor tells you that it will hurt for only a few seconds. You know that you can manage this acute pain—pain that will last only a short time—and you feel relieved.

But what would happen if the sting of that needle wouldn't go away—if you felt that pain constantly, month after month, year after year? That kind of long-term pain, which is called chronic pain, is a problem for many people with serious diseases or injuries.

Taking painkilling medicines is one way to deal with chronic pain, but they can affect someone's ability to think and react. They may produce side effects such as an upset stomach or sleeplessness. And, finally, many painkilling drugs can be addictive. For these reasons, many people are eager for drugless ways of coping with their pain. Medical electricity is a promising alternative.

But electric pain control works only when it is carefully planned and performed by a doctor. Electricity can be extremely dangerous. No one but a medical expert should ever send electricity into anyone's body. Only electricity that is delivered to exactly the right place in the right amounts can help control pain.

Under normal circumstances, pain is useful. It lets you to know when tissue in a certain part of your body—the part where you feel the pain—is being damaged. For example, if you used a bare hand to take a hot, metal-handled pan from a stove, you would feel a sharp burning pain in your hand. To make you drop the pan and avoid seriously injuring your hand, your body's nervous system would go into immediate action. The nerves in your hand would send a message to the neurons in your spinal cord. This message, without even reaching your brain, would cause a second message to speed back from your spinal cord to the muscles in

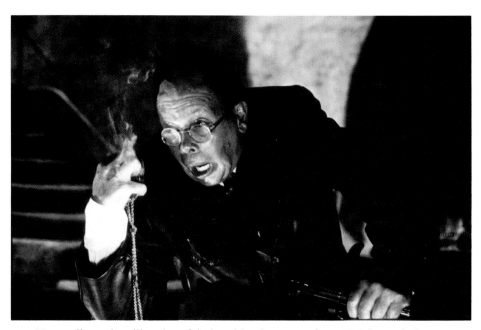

Normally, pain—like that felt by this character from Raiders of the Lost Ark—*puts your nervous system into immediate action.*

your hand. As a result, you'd immediately drop the pan. This reaction is good. Acute pain—from a burn, a cut, a muscle strain, or any other injury—helps you withdraw quickly from danger.

But when pain is chronic, it loses its purpose as a warning. There is no danger to withdraw from. The pain serves only to remind you of some problem within the body, a problem that you can't escape. Chronic pain can be caused by diseases such as arthritis or cancer or by an injury that takes a long time to heal. Even though such pain might, in its early stages, help doctors locate and diagnose a problem, the pain often lingers far beyond its usefulness. At this point, a patient might start a program of electric pain control.

Endorphins

Why does electrical stimulation of nerves deaden pain? A possible explanation is the endorphin theory. Electrical stimulation causes neurons to produce **endorphins,** the body's natural pain-control chemicals. Scientists who back this theory believe that the most effective way to start endorphin production is to send short bursts of mild electricity to nerve cells in the spinal cord or the brain. The body responds to the electricity by producing endorphins, which settle in the pain-control centers in the brain. There the endorphins stop the brain from processing pain messages. If the endorphin theory is true, electrical therapy clearly can reduce pain—and has done so for many patients.

Applying the Current

An early method of electrically treating pain had a relationship to acupuncture—an ancient way of treating sick people by inserting needles into special locations in the body. Even though acupuncture was developed in China, European doctors were aware

63

of this treatment. A French doctor named L. V. J. Berlioz first suggested in 1816 that the needles used in acupuncture could be connected to an electrical machine for the treatment of pain. At that time, the electrodes used in electrical therapy were placed on the skin. To get the current past the skin and into the body, doctors had to use high-powered current, which caused painful skin burns. Berlioz believed that, by inserting needles directly into muscles and nerves, doctors could bypass the skin's natural resistance to electricity. A lower-powered current could then be used, thereby avoiding skin burns.

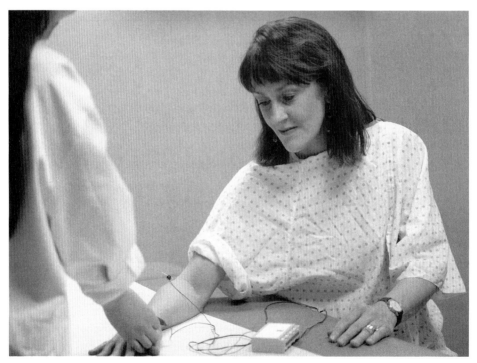

A low-powered electrical current—inserted directly to muscles and nerves with acupuncture needles—relieves chronic pain.

Surface electrodes are placed on the skin.

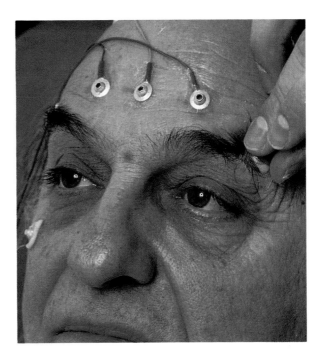

In modern pain treatments, two types of electrodes are used: surface electrodes (placed on the skin) and implanted electrodes (placed beneath the skin to stimulate nerve cells directly). Surface electrodes are much improved over those used in Berlioz's time. Lubricated by gels, they make smoother contact with the skin and more evenly distribute power through the contact surface of the electrode. These improvements—and better safety procedures— have eliminated the problem of skin burns from surface electrodes. Implanted electrodes do not have much in common with Berlioz's electrified needles, except that they deliver current to tissues deeper than the skin. Put into place by surgeons, implanted electrodes are meant to stay for a long time where they have been installed—in muscle, the spinal cord, or even the brain.

The most common modern way of sending painkilling electricity to nerves is with a small machine known as a **transcutaneous electrical nerve stimulator,** or TENS unit. (Cutaneous refers to skin; transcutaneous means "across the skin.") A TENS device uses two surface electrodes—one positive and one negative—so that the current can pass through a specific part of the body from one electrode to the other. This keeps the electricity concentrated where

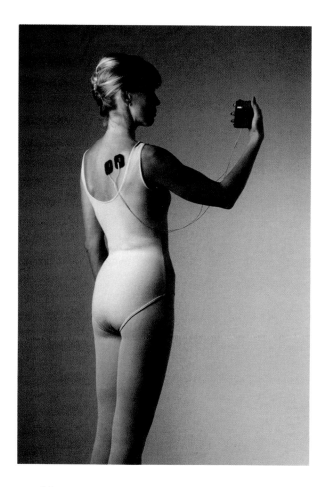

The electrical pulses from a TENS unit feel like tingling taps.

it is needed. A cable leads from each electrode to a boxlike central unit. This contains a power supply and has controls for adjusting the power level and the pulse rate (the number of electrical signals per minute). In a typical treatment routine, a TENS unit will deliver 80 to 100 pulses each minute for 15 to 45 minutes, three times a day.

Patients report that they feel a quick, tingling tap with each pulse of electricity. For some, this is uncomfortable or even painful. A pain-control system that causes new pain is not beneficial, so the power and pulse rate have to be lowered to make the treatment tolerable. Other patients need the power level higher. If it is set too high, however, it might make the muscles in the area of the electrode contract uncontrollably. Usually, the power level and pulse rate are set just above the tingling point. At this level, they are effective but still too mild to make the muscles contract.

Since a TENS system must stimulate specific nerves, the placement of the electrodes is important. But sometimes the electrodes, even after they have been properly placed, must be moved. Many patients report that, after several weeks of TENS treatment, their electrical therapy is less effective. Through a process that researchers still don't understand, the nerves seem to adapt gradually to electrical stimulation, and this makes them less responsive to the pain treatment. If the electrodes are moved slightly, however, they can stimulate a new set of nerves in the painful area, giving renewed relief from pain.

Many TENS units are small enough to be clipped to a belt. By carrying the TENS system like a miniature CD player, a patient with arthritis, cancer, or low back pain can continue normal daily activities and not go to the doctor's office every day for pain therapy. However, the patient must remember to take the TENS unit off before taking a bath or going for a swim.

Direct to the Brain

Because the brain plays a key role in processing the body's pain signals, it was natural for researchers to ask: What would happen if you applied electricity directly to the brain? As dangerous as this sounds, it can relieve pain. Still, because so little is known about how the brain's pain-processing system works, direct stimulation of the brain is used only when nothing else has relieved the pain.

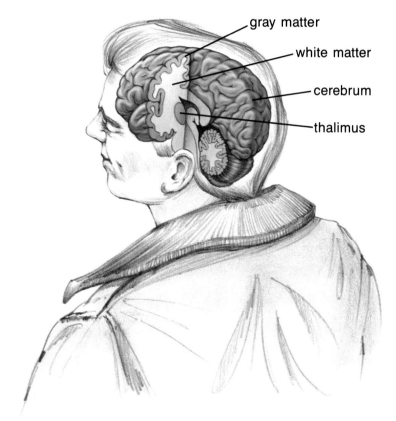

A cross-section of the brain shows the thalamic region and the cerebrum's white and gray matter.

Electrical stimulation has successfully controlled pain in two areas of the brain. One area is in the cerebrum, and the other is in the thalamic region in the center of the brain. The cerebrum, the top part of the brain, has a large surface area full of folds and indentations. The outside of the cerebrum is the well-known gray matter of the brain; the inside is known as the white matter. The gray matter of the cerebrum first receives sensory information, including pain signals, from the rest of the body. This information is then sent to the white matter, where it is processed and acted upon. The best site in the cerebrum for electrical pain therapy is the gray matter, where electricity can block the pain signals before they are sent on for further processing.

When electrical stimulators are implanted in the brain, setting the power level and stimulation time is especially crucial—and especially tricky. A brain stimulator is implanted in the patient's skull and cannot be easily adjusted later. These units are battery-powered, and replacement of the battery involves surgery. To lengthen battery life, doctors must set the power and stimulation times at the lowest level that can still control the pain. Making these fine adjustments is very difficult because the patient does not feel any tingling sensation in the brain that could let the doctor know when the stimulation has reached some basic level.

The success rate for electrical stimulation of the brain is quite good immediately after the implantation surgery. However, many patients report that the pain returns, sometimes years later. Further research into electrical brain stimulation should lead to more precise stimulators with longer-lasting effectiveness. A greater understanding of the brain's role in pain perception will probably also increase the effectiveness of TENS units. Encouraged by the progress that has already made electricity valuable in pain control, medical researchers see high potential in this line of research.

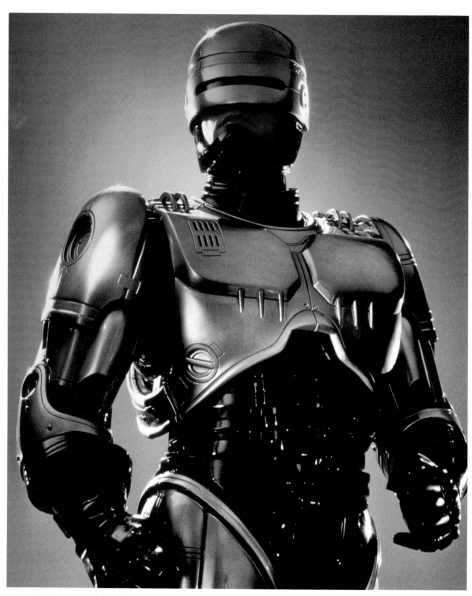

With the aid of electrical stimulations, the fictional Robocop has super-sensitive ears.

70

CHAPTER
6

FUTURE SHOCKS

Medical electricity has proven itself. Treating ailments by sending electric current directly into the human body no longer seems like a lunatic idea out of science fiction. But the full range of possibilities for medical electricity has yet to be discovered. Beyond the relatively established uses—cardiac pacing and defibrillation, muscle stimulation, and pain management—newer, more experimental applications are being explored. Some of these, real as they are, still sound a lot like science fiction.

The Deaf Hear

Some intriguing, though exaggerated, hints about electricity's ability to restore hearing come from fictional characters, such as television's Six Million Dollar Man and RoboCop. Advanced electronics gave these characters super-sensitive ears that could hear a human voice clear across town. New developments in electrical stimulation of hearing cannot go that far, but electronic applications can help the deaf to hear. For a person who hasn't heard a human voice in many years, being able suddenly to hear is no less amazing than RoboCop's ability to eavesdrop from half a mile away.

Electrically stimulated hearing is possible because the brain receives sound messages as electrical impulses. Sound is a type of energy that travels in waves. The distance between the crest, or top, of one wave and the top of the next determines the pitch of the sound: Long sound waves are heard as low pitches and short sound waves as high pitches. The number of sound waves that go by in one second determine that sound's frequency. The human ear can detect sound only within a certain range of frequencies—from 20 to 20,000 waves per second. These are the sounds that the ear is able to translate from sound waves into electrical messages for the brain.

The ear is made up of three parts: the outer ear, the middle ear, and the inner ear. The outer ear, the part that we can see, funnels sound into the middle ear. The middle ear is made up of the tympanic membrane, or ear drum, and three tiny bones (the smallest bones in the body) connected together in a chain. When sound enters the middle ear, the tympanic membrane vibrates. The membrane is connected to the chain of three bones, and they, too, vibrate. At the innermost end of the chain of bones is another membrane called the oval window. This is the entrance to the inner ear.

On the inner side of the oval window is a liquid-filled chamber called the cochlea. It is a long, narrow chamber coiled up into the shape of a snail's shell. When the oval-window membrane moves back and forth, it sends waves through the liquid in this chamber, much like the waves made by moving your hand back and forth through bathwater. Lining the cochlea are special hair cells that move in response to certain waves. This movement stimulates nerve cells attached to the hair cells. That stimulation starts an electrical signal that travels, through a bundle of neurons called the auditory nerve, to the brain for analysis. Each hair is tuned to a specific frequency, moving only in response to waves

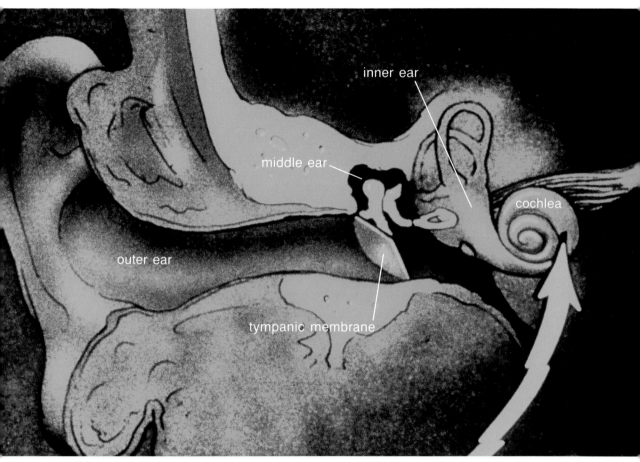

Each hair inside the inner ear's cochlea, shown here, is tuned to a different frequency.

of that frequency. One end of the cochlea has the hairs that respond to low sounds, and the other has those that respond to high ones.

If any part of your ear is not working, you will not hear normally. Damage to the middle ear can be repaired by surgery. Some

73

inner-ear problems can be alleviated by hearing aids, which make sounds louder. But sometimes the hair cells in the inner ear are badly damaged or destroyed. When this happens, the neurons that are supposed to be stimulated by the hair cells stop sending signals to the brain. But, since neurons can be stimulated electrically, electric current can sometimes do the job that is ordinarily done by the hair cells. Electricity itself, not stimulation from the hair cells, can cause the nerve cells to pass messages about sounds to the

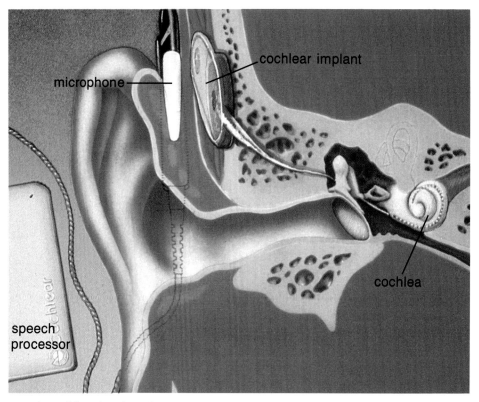

A cochlear implant bypasses damaged hair cells and stimulates nerves to pass sound messages to the brain.

74

brain. Electrical stimulation of these nerve cells can be accomplished with a device called a cochlear implant.

The first experimental cochlear stimulators were surgically implanted in 1972. This type of implant became possible only with the development of very tiny electrodes that pick up a signal from a microphone outside the body. The cochlea is only the size of a quarter, and thousands of nerve cells have contact points along this small part of the ear. Only a minuscule, very flexible electrode could isolate and stimulate several of the nerve-connection spots along the cochlea. By the 1970s, the same technology used in producing minute parts for computers had produced tiny electrodes, some with lead wires 10 times thinner than a human hair. Each miniaturized implant can have as many as 20 leads, and each lead could stimulate one nerve connection.

A cochlear-implant system receives sound through a microphone in the user's ear, but these sounds are not transmitted directly to the nerves in the ear. Instead, they go first to a small portable computer, probably hanging on the user's belt, that can strengthen the most important parts of the sounds. The computer then sends electrical messages to a receiver in the user's skull, and this receiver passes the messages to electrodes in the user's cochlea. By stimulating the neurons that feed into the auditory nerve, these electrodes send messages about sounds to the brain.

It is impossible to implant enough electrodes to stimulate each one of the thousands of nerve endings in the cochlea. Therefore, people with cochlear implants cannot hear as many sounds as people with unimpaired hearing can. Still, implants do help a lot of people hear bells, cars, and trucks—important sounds for anyone planning to cross a street—and pleasant sounds like the rhythmic patterns in music, a friend's voice, or a bird chirping. A 1992 story in the Minneapolis *StarTribune* told of one 10-year-old recipient of a $30,000 cochlear implant who was surprised to learn that flushing toilets make noise. "It's a noisy world," she said. Cochlear implants have become sophisticated enough to help many deaf people hear and understand voices—even by telephone.

Implants are not equally successful for all deaf people. Fewer than 20 percent of people with cochlear implants can hear voices well enough to understand them, but most people with implants either hear voices in only a fuzzy way or not at all. People who have lost their hearing before learning to speak cannot learn spoken language with only the aid of a cochlear implant.

People whose auditory nerves have been damaged cannot benefit at all from a cochlear implant, because the implant system depends on being able to send electrical signals to the brain by way of a healthy auditory nerve. For people with auditory nerve damage, a different type of implant that directly stimulates the brain is the only kind of technology that might create hearing. Although some such implants have been designed, they create only the crudest type of hearing and are not yet available to the public.

All of this technology is expensive, and it can't help everyone. Until vast improvements can be made in cochlear implants and direct stimulators of the brain, most of the hearing impaired and their families will continue to rely on sign language and other forms of voiceless communication. Still, cochlear implants have already helped thousands of people hear at least some sounds again. The prospects seem good for steady improvement in this technology, and cochlear implants should become more affordable as they become more common.

And the Blind See

In the science-fiction television show *Star Trek: The Next Generation,* a character named Lt. Geordi La Forge, blind from birth,

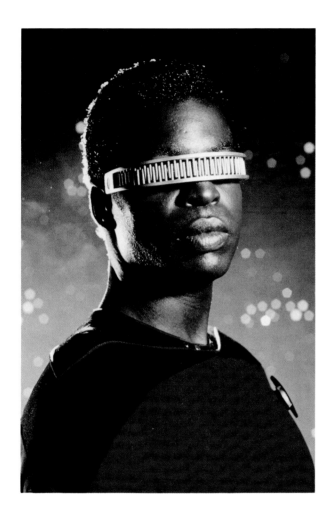

Star Trek's *character* *Geordi La Forge can* *see with the help of* *a visor that stimulates* *his nerves.*

wears a light-sensing visor that stimulates his sight nerves. Perfect artificial sight for the blind has not become a reality, but some advances in electrically stimulated sight have occurred.

Before World War II, researchers discovered that a blind patient could detect a spot of light if a certain part of the brain, the visual cortex, was electrically stimulated. When doctors stimulated one

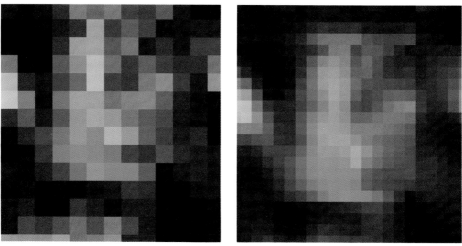

With only a few electrodes to stimulate sight, an image would be hard to make out, figure 1. *With progressively more information*

site in the visual cortex and then another, the patient reported that the spot of light changed location. These early experiments suggested that sending power to some of the electrodes in a grid— an arrangement of rows and columns like the squares on a chessboard—might create a pattern of light that a blind person would see as a recognizable shape. Experiments in the 1960s and 1970s in England and the United States confirmed that an electrode grid could help blind patients to see arrangements of light.

Still, a number of problems arose. The first problem was how to arrange the electrodes. No direct relationship could be found between the arrangement of electrodes in the visual cortex and the location at which the patient saw the spot of light. One electrode placed to the right of another did not necessarily create a spot of light to the right of the first spot. Another problem was the size of the equipment. The electrodes needed for electrical

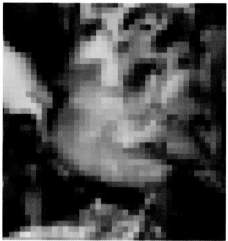 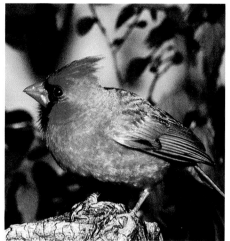

stimulating our sight nerves, figures 2, 3, *and* 4, *we can see finer and finer details.*

stimulation of sight would have to be even smaller than those used in a cochlear implant. To create a visual-stimulation grid, a huge number of very small electrodes are necessary. Even a very simple grid of 10 electrodes across and 10 down would require 100 electrodes. Each of these must be far enough away from the others to prevent its neighbors from flashing on every time it generated a signal.

To understand the difficulty of creating an image with dots of light, try drawing a simple picture—say, a house—by making dots on a piece of paper. The greater the number of dots in your picture, the clearer that picture will be. You can imagine then how many dots are needed to create even very basic vision. Electrical sight stimulation demands as many individual stimulation points as possible. If lots of electrodes are in the brain, however, the chances are great that one might accidently stimulate others.

A research team led by Professor Richard Normann at the University of Utah has developed a grid of electrodes that might overcome this problem. Earlier experiments used surface electrodes, but these new electrodes can be inserted deeper into the brain tissue. Needing lower power to work, these internal electrodes are less likely to stimulate one another accidentally. To further reduce this possibility, the electrodes in the grid are arranged so that each row of electrodes reaches deeper into the brain than the one before it. As many as 100 electrodes can be crowded onto the grid without their tips getting close enough to interfere with one another.

Even so, there is the arrangement problem—the fact that two electrodes side by side in the brain do not necessarily produce side-by-side spots of light. The vision-stimulation sites in the brain will have to be carefully identified and mapped out. Then, computer programs will have to be developed to make incoming light stimulate the proper electrodes and create a meaningful pattern of light spots.

Electrically stimulated sight, despite recent progress, is a long way off. No one can do more than guess at how such a system would work. In theory, a camera would probably be worn, like glasses, at the front of the head. The light from the camera would be processed into electrical impulses, and a computer would determine which impulse should go to which electrode. The signal would be transmitted through wires to the electrodes, which would then stimulate the visual cortex.

Although these new electrodes might help patients recognize patterns around them, the vision that they may produce is likely to be rather elementary. Since the grid of electrodes is small, the field of vision will be narrow. Someone with an implanted grid will only be able to see things that are directly ahead, as if the world were perpetually seen through a tunnel. Objects too far to the side of where the user is looking would be invisible, because the grid doesn't contain enough electrodes to represent them.

A different kind of electrical implant may someday help patients whose eyes have been damaged but who still have healthy optic nerves—nerves leading from the eye to the brain. A retinal implant, an electrical device planted in the eye, might be able to take in light, translate it into electrical signals, and then pass these messages to the visual cortex by way of the optic nerve.

No real vision has yet been created by medical electricity. Researchers still struggle with very difficult problems involving the technology. Even if implants in the visual cortex or the retina do someday become common, they might help blind people read very slowly—much more slowly than with the Braille system of reading by touch. But, slow as this reading might be, non-Braille materials such as street signs and notices on bulletin boards would become accessible to blind people. Artificial sight would probably also be good enough to help blind people move around large objects. The possibilities for this type of medical electricity are encouraging, and *Star Trek's* Geordi La Forge may indeed have real-life counterparts someday.

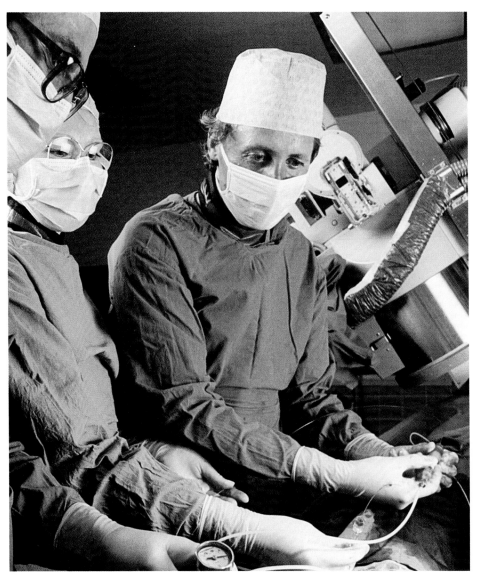

Through years of research, scientists have found ways for medical electricity to make our lives better. Today, when someone's heart beats irregularly, implanting a pacemaker is routine.

82

NEW PATHWAYS

Some possible medical applications of electrical current are even farther out on the frontiers of medicine. For example, electrical stimulation of one of the nerves in the brain, the vagus nerve, is being tried as a way to treat epilepsy—a condition in which someone has occasional episodes of falling and uncontrolled movement that might cause serious injury to himself or herself.

There is evidence that wounds and broken bones heal faster when electrical stimulation is applied. Electricity could even be used in birth control. Scientists are working on a contraceptive device that, implanted in a woman's body, could use electrical shocks to repel sperm cells before they can reach the egg cell.

Electricity may also become a weapon in the battle against AIDS. A research team headed by William D. Lyman at the Albert Einstein College of Medicine in New York City recently discovered that exposing an AIDS-causing virus to low-voltage electricity greatly reduces its ability to infect human white blood cells. The research showed that the shocked viruses lost the ability to make a critical enzyme that enables them to reproduce in the white blood cells. For patients already infected, blood might be pumped out of the body, treated with an electrical current, and then returned to the body.

Medical electricity, promising as it is, develops only through careful, expensive research. Still, with a history of great successes in cardiac pacing and defibrillation, muscle stimulation, and pain control, medical electricity seems well worth the investment.

Glossary

asynchronous pacing—a type of heart pacing in which the pacemaker sends out an electrical pulse whether the heart needs it or not. Asynchronous pacing keeps the heart beating at the same speed all the time, without changing the speed of the heartbeat to match the body's activity.

atrioventricular (AV) node—a part of the heart that picks up messages from the sinoatrial node and passes them along to the ventricles

atrium—one of the heart's two upper chambers. One atrium receives oxygen-rich blood from the lungs and pumps it into a ventricle. The other atrium receives oxygen-poor blood from the rest of the body and pumps it into the other ventricle.

axon—the long, narrow extension of a neuron that carries charges away from the cell body toward muscles, glands, or other neurons.

defibrillator—a machine that stops the heart's ventricles from fluttering uncontrollably

demand pacing—a type of heart pacing in which the pacemaker sends out a signal only when the heart has trouble timing the heartbeat on its own

dendrite—one of the many branches that extend from the body of a neuron that pick up signals from other neurons

electric current—a charge that moves in a definite direction

endorphin—a pain-control chemical made by the human body

functional electrical stimulation (FES)—electrical current that, when applied to the human body, helps part of the body to function

functional neuromuscular stimulation (FNS)—a type of functional electrical stimulation in which electricity is sent through the nerves to help muscles function

ion—an atom that has an electrical charge because it has gained or lost electrons

medical electricity—electricity sent into some part of the human body to treat illness or injury, to relieve pain, or to help some part of the body function

membrane—a thin covering that surrounds a cell

neuron—a nerve cell

neurotransmitters—the chemicals that jump the synapse between neurons to transmit a message

pacemaker—a machine that helps a heart to keep beating at the proper speed

rate-responsive pacemaker—a pacemaker that senses the body's level of activity and causes the heart to beat at different speeds at different times to match that activity

sinoatrial (SA) node—a group of cells in the right atrium. The SA node generates electrical signals that tell the heart how fast to beat.

spinal cord—a bundle of neurons that extends down the back from the base of the brain to just above the waist. The spinal cord is enclosed in the hollow bones of the backbone, or spine.

synapse—the small gap between the axon of one neuron and the dendrite of another

transcutaneous electrical nerve stimulator (TENS)—a device that sends painkilling electricity through the skin to reach the nerves below the skin's surface

ventricle—one of the two lower chambers of the heart. One ventricle pumps oxygen-poor blood out to the lungs. The other pumps oxygen-rich blood out to the rest of the body.

ventricular fibrillation—a condition in which the ventricles stop pumping and begin fluttering uncontrollably

Index

Marsolais, Dr. E. Byron, 56, 57
medical electricity, definition of, 8, 85
membrane, 14–15, 17–18, 85
muscle, 17–18, 19, 48, 49, 50, 51–52, 53–59, 65
muscle-stimulation system, electrical, 54–59, 84

negative ions, 12–14, 15
nervous system, 50
neuron, 10, 13–17, 19, 20, 21, 51, 56, 62, 63, 72, 73, 85
neurotransmitters, 16–17, 85

pacemaker, 9, 30, 33, 85; externally powered, 33, 35–36; implanted, 39, 40, 41–44, 82; self-powered, external, 37–39. *See also* asynchronous pacing, demand pacing, rate-responsive pacemaker
pain. *See* acute pain, chronic pain
paralysis, 9, 50, 52–53. *See also* paraplegia, quadriplegia
paraplegia, 48, 52, 54, 55, 56
positive ions, 12–15, 17–18
proton, 11–12
pulse generator, 41–44

quacks, medical, 27–29
quadriplegia, 52, 55, 56–57

rate-responsive pacemaker, 41, 85
reflex motion, 19, 20, 62

septum, 34–35
sight, electrical stimulation of, 9, 77–81
sinoatrial (SA) node, 19, 32, 33, 34, 44, 85

skeletal muscle. *See* muscle
smooth muscle. *See* muscle
sodium ions. *See* positive ions
spinal cord, 13, 19, 20, 21, 50, 51, 62, 65, 85
spinal-cord injury, 50, 52–54
static electricity, 23
synapse, 16, 85

thalimus, 68, 69
transcutaneous electrical nerve stimulator (TENS), 66–67, 69, 85

ventricle, 32, 34, 44, 45, 85
ventricular fibrillation, 45, 46, 47, 85
vertebrae, 50, 52
visual cortex, 77–78, 80, 81
Volta, Alessandro, 25

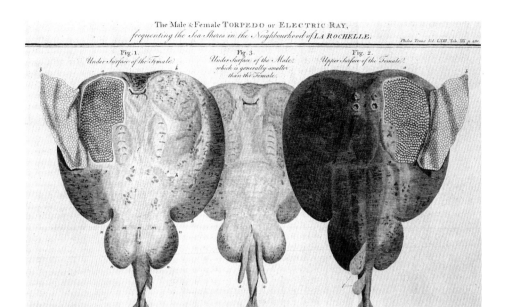

The Male & Female TORPEDO or ELECTRIC RAY, *frequenting the Sea Shores in the Neighbourhood of LA ROCHELLE.*

Phil. Trans. Vol. LXIII Tab. XIX p. 490

Fig. 1. *Under Surface of the Female.*

Fig. 3. *Under Surface of the Male, which is generally smaller than the Female.*

Fig. 2. *Upper Surface of the Female.*

Photo Acknowledgments

Photographs and illustrations reproduced with the permission of: Marquette Electronics, pp. 2, 46 (top); Hollywood Book and Poster, pp. 6, 62, 70, 77; Visuals Unlimited/© SIU, pp. 8, 46 (bottom), 65; Visuals Unlimited/© Triarch Visuals Unlimited, p. 10; Brian Liedahl, pp. 12, 15, 16, 20, 21, 34, 35, 42, 51, 68; Visuals Unlimited/© David M. Phillips, pp. 14, 18; The Bakken Library and Museum, Minneapolis, pp. 22, 25, 26, 28, 88; Science Visuals Unlimited/Cardiac Control Systems, p. 30; University of Minnesota Archives, p. 36; Medtronic, Inc., pp. 37, 38, 40, 43, 82; Catherine Manderfield, p. 39; Kathy Goodstein/Shiners Hospitals—Philadelphia Unit, pp. 48, 58; Cleveland FES Center, p. 52; Adrian Kantrowitz, M.D., Surgical Resources Lab, Detroit, MI, p. 54; Sigmedics, Inc., p. 55; Dr. E. Byron Marsolais, p. 57; Empi, Inc., pp. 60, 66; Nancy Leegard/Acupuncture and Alternative Medicine, HCMC, p. 64; Cochlear Corporation, pp. 73, 74; Perry J. Reynold, pp. 78, 79.

Cover photographs reproduced with the permission of: Marquette Electronics, front; Empi, Inc., back; Visuals Unlimited/© David M. Phillips, background.